Cultural And Interfaith Relationships

The Tapestry of Cultural and Interfaith Unity

John Dollar

Copyright © 2023

by

John dollar

Table of Contents

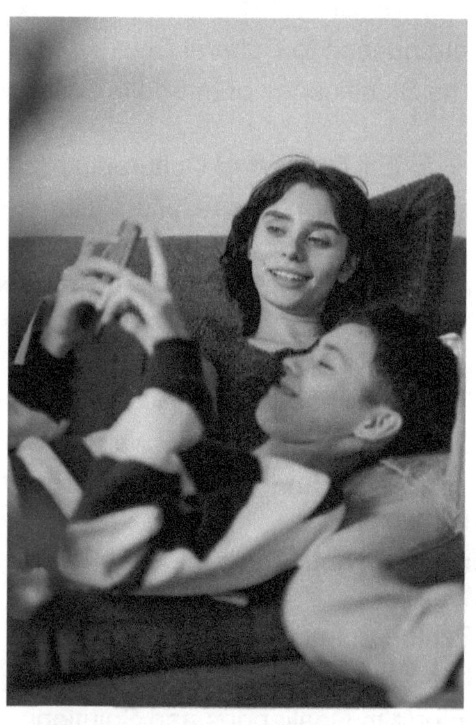

INTRODUCTION

In the vibrant city of Harmonyville, where different cultures and faiths coexisted, lived Maya, a young artist with a penchant for breaking social norms. With her radiant spirit, Maya found herself drawn to the enchanting melodies of the Sufi mystics, even though her roots were deeply rooted in the traditions of her Hindu upbringing.

One day, as the sun sank below the horizon, Maya's art studio became a haven for creative souls from various walks of life. Among them was Zayn, a thoughtful poet whose verses resonated with the wisdom of various religious philosophies. Maya and Zayn, despite their different backgrounds, discovered a common appreciation for the tapestry of human experience woven through cultural and spiritual diversity.

Their friendship blossomed and transcended the boundaries set by societal expectations. They often found themselves engaged in conversations that delved into the rich tapestry of their respective heritages. From vibrant Holi festivals to soulful rituals of Sufi gatherings, Maya and Zayn celebrated the beauty of their differences.

As their bond deepened, Maya's parents, traditionalists rooted in their Hindu faith, could not understand the connection between their daughter and Zayn. The once harmonious family dynamic was strained by fears of social judgments and fear of cultural dilution. The clash between tradition and modernity reflected the struggles faced by many in Harmonyville.

Determined to bridge the gap between generations and beliefs, Maya initiated a gathering in her home, inviting friends and family to openly share their cultural and religious practices. The living room was transformed into a kaleidoscope of colors, scents and melodies as each guest contributed a piece of their heritage. Zayn, with his eloquent verses, became the thread that weaved these diverse elements into a harmonious symphony.

In the midst of a lively celebration, Maya's parents witnessed the beauty that emerged when different traditions came together. Barriers of misunderstanding collapsed as shared laughter and the aroma of different cuisines filled the air. Maya's parents slowly began to recognize the strength in unity and understood that embracing diversity did not diminish their own cultural identity.

Maya and Zayn's love story flourished in this cultural exchange, drawing inspiration from the acceptance and understanding that surrounded them. However, the journey was not without problems. Outside pressures from conservative corners of Harmonyville sought to impose rigid norms on the unconventional couple. The love that blossomed between Maya and Zayn faced trials that mirrored the struggles of countless interfaith relationships. Undeterred, Maya and Zayn decide to embark on a journey that will take them to the roots of their respective cultures. They traveled to an ancestral Mayan village where ancient chants echoed through the air and the soil whispered stories of generations past. Here Zayn experienced the essence of Hindu traditions, understood the cultural nuances that shaped Maya's worldview.

In return, Maya accompanied Zayn to the mystical lands that inspired his poetic verses. For her, dervish dances and Sufi rituals became a deep exploration of spirituality, shattering preconceived notions and fostering a deeper connection with universal truths that transcend religious boundaries.

Their journey became a testimony to the transformative power of love and understanding. As Maya and Zayn returned to Harmonyville, they carried with them the wisdom gained from exploring each other's worlds. They became advocates of cultural and interfaith harmony and inspired others in their community with their experiences.

Ultimately, Harmonyville lived up to its name as it embraced the love between Maya and Zayn and realized that unity in diversity is not just a slogan but a living, breathing reality. The couple's journey lit the way for others, proving that the intermingling of cultures and faiths can create a mosaic of beauty, strength and resilience.

And so, in the heart of Harmonyville, Maya and Zayn continued to nurture their love, surrounded by a community that had learned to appreciate the rich tapestry of human connection, crossing the lines of culture and faith.

Cultural and interfaith relations represent a fascinating intersection of different backgrounds, beliefs and traditions. In an increasingly interconnected world, individuals from different cultural and religious backgrounds find themselves in complex relationships that transcend the boundaries of their heritage. These volumes bring a rich tapestry of experiences, challenges and opportunities for growth. In this survey, we delve into the dynamics of cultural and interfaith relationships, exploring the nuances that shape these connections and the ways in which individuals navigate the delicate balance between maintaining their cultural and religious identities while creating a shared life with a partner from another country. Background.

At the heart of cultural and interreligious relations lies the fusion of different traditions and values. Whether celebrating cultural holidays, observing religious rituals, or passing down ancestral customs, these relationships often require embracing diversity. Couples are immersed in a lively exchange of ideas, customs and practices, creating a unique blend that reflects the mosaic of their combined identities. This fusion is not without challenges, as the partners must negotiate differences and find common ground in their shared aspirations while respecting the individual roots from which they spring.

One of the key dynamics at play in cultural and interreligious relations is the negotiation of religious beliefs. Individuals entering into these relationships may come from faiths with different doctrines, traditions, and interpretations of spirituality. The interplay between religious differences can be both rewarding and complex, requiring open communication, mutual understanding and a willingness to engage in respectful dialogue. Navigating the complexities of shared religious practices, raising children of dual cultural or religious heritage, and finding common ground on matters of faith are all aspects that require careful consideration and compromise.

Moreover, cultural and interfaith relations often act as a microcosm of broader societal dynamics, reflecting ongoing dialogue about diversity, inclusion and acceptance. These relationships challenge social norms and offer a glimpse into a world where love transcends the boundaries of ethnicity, nationality and religion. They thus contribute to the wider discourse on multiculturalism and pluralism and argue for a more inclusive understanding of what constitutes a traditional relationship.

Despite the potential for growth and enrichment, cultural and interfaith relationships can encounter external pressures and societal prejudices. Discrimination, stereotyping, and misconceptions can occur, placing additional burdens on couples navigating these unions. This requires resilience and a shared commitment to overcoming social barriers, fostering a sense of unity that transcends the external judgments that may be placed upon them.

Family dynamics also come into play, as cultural and interfaith relationships may face varying degrees of acceptance within extended families. Bridging the gap between generations, each rooted in a different cultural or religious context, can be a delicate process. The challenge is to foster understanding and appreciation among family members who may have deeply held beliefs about tradition and heritage. Successfully navigating these challenges often involves open communication, education, and a shared commitment to making connections that transcend cultural and religious differences.

Indeed, communication proves to be a fundamental pillar of the success of cultural and interreligious relations. The ability to articulate your values, expectations and concerns while actively listening to your partner's point of view is paramount. This ongoing dialogue allows couples to proactively address potential conflicts and fosters an environment of mutual respect and understanding. It also provides an opportunity for couples to celebrate their differences and find joy in the shared aspects of their unique journey.

Education and exposure play a key role in promoting understanding within cultural and interfaith relationships. Couples often embark on a journey of discovery, getting to know each other's backgrounds, histories and social contexts that have shaped their identities. This process of mutual discovery serves not only to deepen their connection, but also to cultivate a broader awareness of the world around them. Exposure to different cultural practices and religious traditions can lead to a more enriched and empathetic perspective, breaking down stereotypes and fostering a true appreciation of diversity.

Cultural and interreligious relations form a fascinating tapestry woven from threads of different traditions, beliefs and identities. While these relationships present unique challenges, they also offer unique opportunities for growth, understanding, and connection. By navigating the complexities of cultural and religious differences with open communication, respect, and a shared commitment to creating a unique identity, couples can build lasting foundations that celebrate the richness of diversity. In doing so, they contribute to a larger narrative of a world where love knows no borders and where relationships serve as powerful catalysts for unity in an ever evolving global landscape.

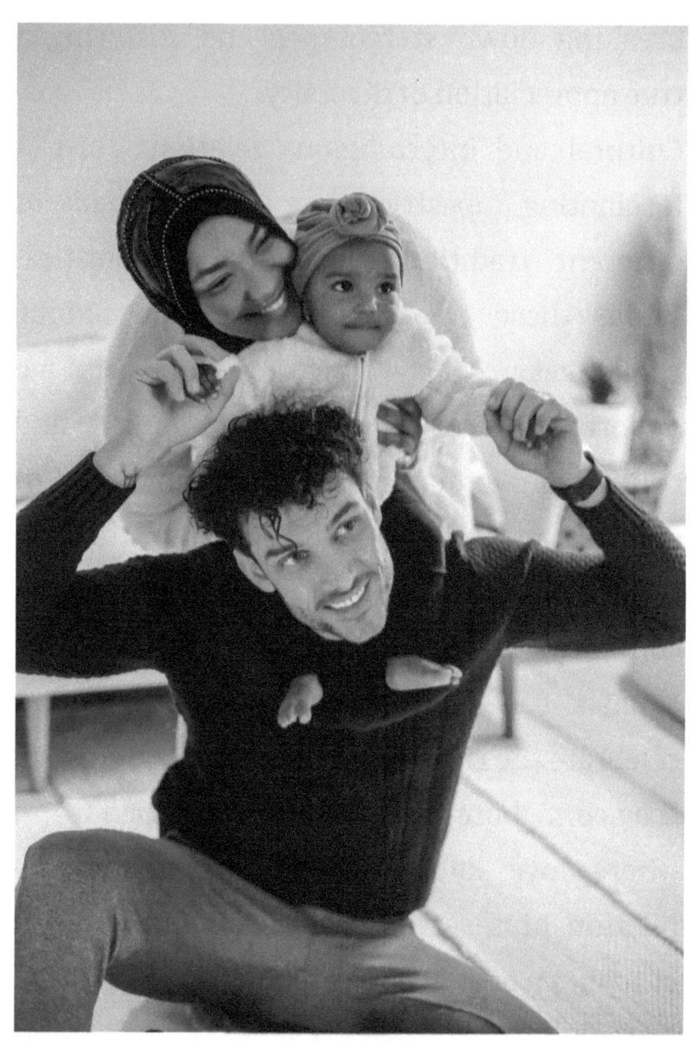

Chapter 1: Foundations of Cultural and Interfaith Understanding

In our increasingly interconnected world, fostering cultural and interfaith understanding is paramount to building harmonious relationships. The foundations of such understanding lie in a multifaceted approach involving education, empathy, open communication and recognition of shared values. This essay explores the critical components that contribute to the development of cultural and interfaith understanding and highlights their importance in maintaining meaningful relationships.

Education as a cornerstone:
Education plays a key role in laying the foundations for cultural and interfaith understanding. By

providing individuals with insight into different cultures and religions, educational institutions contribute to breaking down stereotypes and dispelling misconceptions. Incorporating multicultural curricula into schools and universities not only broadens students' horizons, but also instills a sense of respect for cultural and religious diversity.

Additionally, educational programs should promote critical thinking and promote dialogue that transcends surface-level differences. This includes examining the historical context, social norms and contribution of different cultures and beliefs to human civilization. By fostering comprehensive understanding, education becomes a powerful tool for bridging divides and cultivating a sense of unity in the midst of diversity.

Empathy as a bridge:

Empathy is a fundamental element in the foundations of cultural and interreligious understanding. It involves stepping into the shoes of others, embracing their experiences, and acknowledging the validity of their perspectives.

Cultivating empathy requires active listening and a willingness to appreciate the emotional and cultural nuances that shape individuals' worldviews.

Through empathy, individuals can overcome cultural and religious barriers and form connections based on shared human experiences. This emotional intelligence fosters a sense of solidarity and reinforces the idea that despite our diverse backgrounds, there is a common thread of humanity that binds us all together.

Open Communication:

Open communication serves as a fundamental pillar for cultural and interfaith understanding. Honest and respectful dialogue allows individuals to express their beliefs, share their stories, and clarify misunderstandings. Creating spaces for open conversations fosters an atmosphere of trust and mutual respect and paves the way for genuine connection.

For example, interfaith dialogues provide a platform for individuals of different faiths to engage in meaningful discussions about their beliefs, practices and values. These dialogues not only increase understanding but also show the similarities that exist between different religious traditions. By emphasizing shared principles, open communication reinforces the idea that common ground can be found even in the midst of apparent differences.

Recognizing Shared Values:
While the recognition and appreciation of cultural and religious differences is essential, the recognition of shared values is equally important. Identifying common ground creates a foundation upon which meaningful relationships can be built. Shared values often cross cultural and religious boundaries and include principles such as compassion, justice and the pursuit of peace.
By focusing on shared values, individuals can find common ground in their aspirations and goals. This shared understanding becomes a unifying force that fosters collaboration and cooperation across diverse cultural and religious backgrounds. It reinforces the idea that despite external differences, there is a shared human essence that binds individuals together.

Challenges and Opportunities:

Despite the importance of cultural and interfaith understanding, challenges remain. Preconceptions, stereotypes and ingrained prejudices can hinder progress. Overcoming these challenges requires continued efforts to remove misconceptions and promote inclusivity.

Opportunities to promote cultural and interfaith understanding may arise through community engagement, cultural exchange programs and collaborative projects. Encouraging individuals to actively participate in these initiatives allows for first-hand experiences that challenge preconceived notions and promote personal growth.

The foundations of cultural and interreligious understanding are essential for building relationships that cross cultural and religious boundaries. Education, empathy, open communication and recognition of shared values form the basis of this understanding. By embracing these foundations, individuals can contribute to a more connected and harmonious world where diversity is celebrated and relationships are built on respect and mutual appreciation.

1.1 Introduction to Cultural Diversity

Cultural diversity is a dynamic and enriching aspect of human society that includes a myriad of traditions, beliefs, languages and practices that shape the identity of individuals and communities. In the context of cultural and interfaith relations, understanding and accepting this diversity is essential to foster mutual respect, harmony and cooperation.

Cultural Diversity Defined:
Cultural diversity refers to the coexistence of different cultural groups within society. These groups may differ in terms of ethnicity, religion, language, customs and values. It is not only about recognizing differences, but also about recognizing the inherent value and contribution of each culture. In an interconnected global landscape, individuals from different cultural backgrounds often find themselves interacting and forming relationships,

making cultural diversity a central theme in today's world.

Importance of Cultural Diversity in Relationships:
In cultural and interreligious relations, the recognition and respect of cultural diversity is paramount. Such relationships connect individuals with different worldviews, traditions and customs. Embracing diversity in these connections promotes openness, tolerance, and a broader perspective on life. It allows individuals to learn from each other and enrich their own cultural experiences.

Challenges in cultural and interreligious relations:
While cultural diversity strengthens relationships, it also presents challenges. Misunderstandings can arise due to different communication styles, values or expectations. Religious differences can add another layer of complexity, which requires patience and empathy to navigate. However, addressing these challenges can lead to stronger, more resilient relationships.

Building cultural competence:

Cultural competence is the ability to understand, appreciate and communicate effectively with people from different cultural backgrounds. In the context of cultural and interfaith relations, building cultural competence is essential to overcoming stereotypes and prejudices. This includes educating yourself about your partner's habits, beliefs, and history, as well as actively listening and engaging in open dialogue.

Supporting Inclusivity:
To create an inclusive environment within cultural and interfaith relations, it is essential to celebrate the uniqueness of each individual while finding common ground. This includes incorporating elements from both cultures into shared experiences such as celebrations, rituals or daily practices. Inclusivity fosters a sense of belonging and unity and reinforces the idea that differences can be a source of strength rather than division.

Benefits of Cultural Diversity in Interfaith Relations:
Cultural diversity brings many advantages to interfaith relations. Exposure to different belief

systems can broaden spiritual understanding and deepen personal growth. It promotes resilience and adaptability as individuals learn to navigate and appreciate different perspectives. Ultimately, such relationships contribute to a more harmonious and interconnected global community.

Educational Initiatives:

Institutions and organizations play a vital role in promoting cultural diversity within relationships. Educational initiatives that focus on intercultural communication, cultural sensitivity and understanding can pave the way for more inclusive societies. Workshops, seminars and awareness campaigns help break down stereotypes and foster an environment where diversity is not only accepted but also celebrated.

In the area of cultural and interfaith relations, embracing cultural diversity is essential to building meaningful connections. It requires a commitment to understanding, respect and continuous learning. By actively engaging and celebrating differences, individuals can create relationships that are not only resilient in the face of challenges, but also contribute to the larger tapestry of a diverse and interconnected world. Through cultural competence, inclusiveness and educational initiatives, we can pave the way for a future where cultural diversity is not only recognized but embraced as a source of strength and unity.

1.2 The Significance of Interfaith Relationships

Interfaith relations are of considerable importance in today's diverse and interconnected world, promoting understanding, tolerance and cultural enrichment. These relationships, where individuals from different religious backgrounds meet, contribute to the tapestry of a global society that thrives on diversity. When examining the meaning of interfaith relationships, it is necessary to delve into the cultural and religious aspects that shape these bonds.

Culturally, interfaith relations play a key role in breaking down barriers and promoting inclusivity. When individuals from different backgrounds come together, they bring unique customs, traditions, and perspectives to their lives together. This intermingling of cultures not only enriches the couple's personal experiences, but also creates a microcosm of cultural exchange that extends into their families and communities. The amalgamation of different practices fosters an environment where mutual respect and recognition of differences flourish.

In addition, interfaith relationships challenge social norms and stereotypes and promote a more open and accepting society. As couples navigate the complexities of merging different cultural elements, they often become ambassadors of understanding and dispel misconceptions about other faiths. This ripple effect contributes to a wider societal shift towards tolerance and appreciation of diversity that transcends religious boundaries.

Religiously, interfaith relationships offer a unique opportunity for dialogue and shared spiritual growth. While differences in religious beliefs may present challenges at first, they also provide a platform for respectful conversations about faith. Couples in interfaith relationships often find common ground in shared values, ethical principles, and commitment to personal and collective growth. This shared journey of exploration and understanding can strengthen the spiritual foundations of a relationship.

Interfaith relations can also serve as a bridge between different religious communities and promote interfaith dialogue at a wider level. The couple becomes a living example of harmony and shows that love and understanding can overcome religious differences. This not only challenges religious prejudices, but also encourages communities to engage in constructive conversations about shared values and goals.

However, it is crucial to be aware of the potential complexities and obstacles that can arise in interfaith relationships. Differences in religious practices, rituals and beliefs can sometimes lead to misunderstandings or conflicts. Effective communication, respect for individual beliefs and a willingness to find common ground become essential ingredients for a successful interfaith relationship.

In coping with these challenges, couples often develop resilience that extends beyond their personal lives. They become advocates of accepting diverse relationships, promoting the idea that love knows no religious boundaries. This advocacy can contribute to social change by encouraging the creation of more inclusive spaces that celebrate diversity rather than stigmatize it.

The importance of interfaith relations lies in their ability to bridge cultural and religious differences and promote a more inclusive and tolerant world. These relationships contribute to the enrichment of cultural tapestries, challenge social norms and provide a platform for constructive dialogue between different religious communities. While we recognize the potential challenges, the transformative power of interfaith relations reaches far beyond the individuals involved, influencing societal attitudes and contributing to the creation of a more harmonious global community.

1.3 Historical Context of Cultural Interactions

Cultural interactions have played a key role in shaping the historical context of human societies, especially in the area of interreligious relations. The dynamic exchange of ideas, beliefs and practices between different cultures has not only enriched civilizations but has also been a source of unity and conflict throughout history.

One of the earliest examples of cultural interactions can be traced back to the Silk Road, a network of trade routes connecting East and West. Various cultures, religions and philosophies intersected along these routes, which encouraged the mutual enrichment of ideas and traditions. The transfer of goods, technology and artistic expressions went hand in hand with the exchange of religious beliefs and cultural practices.

In the Middle Ages, the Iberian Peninsula was a remarkable example of cultural coexistence. During the Islamic rule of Al-Andalus, Christians, Muslims and Jews lived side by side, which contributed to the flourishing of intellectual, scientific and artistic progress. Scholars of various faiths engaged in dialogue, translating ancient Greek and Roman texts, preserving and spreading the knowledge that later fueled the Renaissance in Europe.

However, the Crusades present a contrasting narrative of cultural interactions. These military expeditions aimed at recapturing Jerusalem from the Muslims increased the tension between the Christian and Islamic worlds. While military conflicts dominated, there were instances of cultural exchange where European crusaders adopted aspects of Islamic art, science and governance.

The Renaissance marked a significant period of renewal in Europe, characterized by a renewed interest in classical learning and a human-centered approach to culture. This intellectual movement paved the way for the exploration of other cultures during the Age of Discovery. European powers, driven by economic interests, ventured into distant lands where they clashed with various civilizations in Africa, Asia and the Americas. The cultural exchanges that followed had a profound and lasting impact on global societies.

The colonial era brought complex interactions between colonizers and indigenous cultures. While European powers sought to enforce their values and religions, local traditions influenced aspects of colonial society. The resulting syncretism gave rise to unique cultural manifestations in which both colonizing and colonized elements were mixed.

In more recent history, the 20th century witnessed increased global connectivity that fostered cultural interactions on an unprecedented scale. The rise of mass media, international travel, and communication technology has facilitated the exchange of ideas, pop culture, and religious practices. However, this era also witnessed clashes arising from cultural misunderstandings and geopolitical conflicts.

In particular, interreligious relations have been shaped by historical events and cultural interactions. The religious pluralism of many societies has led to individuals of different faiths coexisting in the same communities. Interfaith dialogue has become essential to foster mutual understanding and respect, especially in regions with a history of religious tension.

The 21st century presents both opportunities and challenges for cultural interactions. Globalization has intensified the interconnectedness of societies, making it imperative for individuals and communities to navigate cultural diversity. However, the same forces that promote interaction also threaten cultural identity, as the homogenizing influence of global trends can erode local traditions.

In conclusion, the historical context of cultural interactions in relation to interfaith relations is a tapestry woven with threads of exchange, conflict and coexistence. From the ancient Silk Road to the challenges of today's globalized world, the interplay of cultures has been the driving force behind shaping human civilization. Recognizing and understanding this complex history is essential to building bridges of understanding and cooperation in our diverse and interconnected world.l

1.4 Importance of Cross-Cultural Competence

Intercultural competence plays a key role in promoting understanding and harmony in different societies, especially in the context of cultural and interreligious relations. In an increasingly interconnected world, individuals and communities must navigate a landscape shaped by a rich tapestry of cultures and religious beliefs. Developing intercultural competence is essential for promoting tolerance, communication and mutual respect, which ultimately contributes to a more harmonious global community.

The basis of intercultural competence is the ability to appreciate and adapt to cultural differences. In the field of cultural relations, this skill goes beyond mere tolerance; it involves an active effort to understand the nuances of different traditions, customs and ways of life. Such understanding forms the basis for building meaningful connections that cross cultural boundaries.

In the context of interreligious relations, intercultural competence acquires another dimension. It requires individuals to navigate complex intersections of religious beliefs, practices, and values. Developing an awareness of different religions and their significance is essential to fostering an atmosphere of respect and acceptance. This competence becomes particularly crucial in societies where multiple religions coexist, as it facilitates dialogue and cooperation while mitigating the potential for religious conflict.

One of the key aspects of intercultural competence is effective communication. Communication is not just about language; it extends to non-verbal cues, gestures and cultural nuances. Misunderstandings can occur when individuals are unaware of the cultural context behind certain expressions or actions. Intercultural competence equips individuals with the skills to interpret and communicate messages effectively, promotes clear communication, and minimizes the risk of unintentional injury.

In addition, intercultural competence promotes empathy by encouraging individuals to step into the shoes of people from different cultural or religious backgrounds. This empathic understanding is the antidote to stereotypes and prejudices that can arise from lack of exposure or familiarity. In interfaith relationships, empathy becomes a bridge between individuals of different religious beliefs, allowing for a deeper appreciation of the spiritual dimensions that shape their lives.

In today's globalized world, businesses, governments and organizations operate on an international scale. Intercultural competence is no longer a desirable trait but a necessity for success. In multicultural workplaces, individuals with cross-cultural competence can easily navigate diverse teams and utilize the strengths that arise from different perspectives. This competency fosters an inclusive environment where everyone feels valued and contributes to common goals.

Cultural intelligence, a key component of intercultural competence, enables individuals to adapt to unfamiliar cultural contexts. This adaptability is vital for individuals involved in interfaith relationships, where encounters with different religious practices and beliefs may require a flexible and open approach. Rather than imposing their own cultural or religious norms, interculturally competent individuals are adept at finding common ground and building connections based on shared values.

In the field of diplomacy and international relations, intercultural competence is a cornerstone for building bridges between peoples with different cultural and religious identities. Understanding the cultural nuances that shape diplomatic interactions is critical to establishing trust and cooperation on the global stage. This competence enables diplomats to navigate sensitive issues with cultural sensitivity and foster diplomatic relations based on mutual respect.

We can say that the importance of intercultural competence in the context of cultural and interreligious relations cannot be overestimated. As the world becomes increasingly interconnected, the ability to navigate and appreciate different cultures and religious beliefs is not just a personal advantage, but a societal imperative. Intercultural competence promotes understanding, effective communication and empathy and lays the foundation for a more inclusive and harmonious global community. Whether in personal relationships, workplaces, or international diplomacy, cultivating intercultural competence is an investment in a more connected and compassionate world.

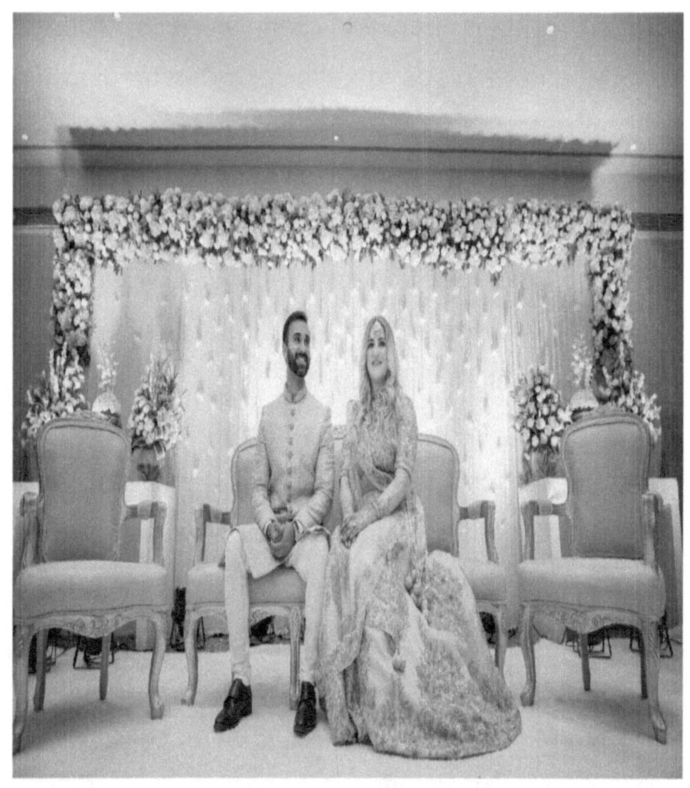

Chapter 2: Navigating Cultural Differences In Relationships

In an increasingly interconnected world, individuals from different cultural and religious backgrounds often find themselves in relationships that cross traditional boundaries. Cultural and interfaith relationships present a unique set of challenges and opportunities that require a delicate balance of understanding, respect and compromise. This article explores the complexities of navigating cultural differences in relationships and focuses on the dynamics within cultural and interfaith contexts.

Understanding Cultural Diversity:
Cultural diversity encompasses a wide range of elements, including language, customs, traditions and values. In the context of relationships, partners from different cultural backgrounds may experience differences in communication styles, family expectations, and social norms. Recognizing and

appreciating these differences is essential to fostering a healthy and harmonious union.

Effective communication:
Communication is the foundation of any successful relationship, and this is especially true in culturally diverse partnerships. Partners must be willing to openly discuss their cultural backgrounds and share insights about their upbringing, beliefs and customs. Active listening becomes the cornerstone that allows each partner to understand and validate the other's perspectives.

Managing expectations:
Cultural expectations often play a significant role in relationships. From family dynamics to societal norms, individuals may carry certain expectations based on their cultural background. It is vital that partners communicate and negotiate these expectations, find common ground and establish shared values that respect both backgrounds.

Respecting traditions:

Cultural and interfaith relationships offer an opportunity to celebrate a rich tapestry of traditions. Instead of viewing differences as obstacles, partners can use the opportunity to learn about and participate in their cultural practices. This not only deepens their connection, but also fosters a sense of inclusion and mutual appreciation.

Navigating Interfaith Challenges:
Interfaith relationships add another layer of complexity because the partners may come from different religious backgrounds with different beliefs and practices. Open and respectful dialogue is essential when dealing with religious differences, allowing couples to explore shared values and find common ground. It is essential to approach these conversations with sensitivity and a willingness to learn.

Building a foundation of shared values:
While cultural and religious differences can be significant, identifying and emphasizing shared values can help bridge the gap. Partners should focus on the principles that bind them together,

such as love, respect and a shared vision for the future. This foundation becomes a guiding force that provides stability in the face of cultural or religious challenges.

How to cope with external pressures:
Intercultural and interfaith couples may face external pressures from family, friends or societal expectations. It is essential to develop strategies for managing these pressures, which may include setting boundaries, educating others about cultural differences, and seeking support from like-minded communities. Building a resilient partnership requires a united front against external challenges.

Celebrating Diversity:
Instead of viewing cultural and interfaith differences as obstacles, couples can choose to celebrate the richness that diversity brings to their relationship. This mindset shift turns challenges into opportunities for growth and mutual understanding. Engaging in joint activities that involve both cultural backgrounds can create a sense of unity and belonging.

Navigating cultural differences in relationships requires patience, empathy, and a commitment to mutual understanding. Cultural and interfaith partnerships offer a unique chance for personal growth and the creation of a rich and varied tapestry of shared experiences. By embracing and celebrating differences, couples can build a resilient foundation that transcends cultural boundaries and foster a relationship that is not only enduring, but enriched by the beauty of diversity.

2.1 Dimensions of Culture

Culture is a multifaceted and dynamic concept that profoundly shapes individuals and societies. When examining cultural and interreligious relations, it is essential to delve into the various dimensions of culture that influence human interactions, beliefs, and values. This exploration helps us understand the complexities and nuances that contribute to the rich tapestry of different societies. In this discussion we will explore the key dimensions of culture and their importance in promoting understanding and harmony in cultural and interfaith relations.

1. Cultural values and norms:

Cultural values serve as the basis for individual and collective behavior in society. They include principles such as individualism or collectivism, power distance, and the importance given to factors such as family, community, and tradition. Understanding and respecting these values is essential in cultural relationships because it shapes expectations and perceptions. In interfaith relations, the recognition of shared and different values between different religious traditions promotes mutual understanding and acceptance.

2. Communication styles:

Communication is the cornerstone of any relationship, and cultural nuances strongly influence how people express themselves. High-context cultures, where communication is implicit and relies on shared context, are different from low-context cultures, which value explicit and direct communication. Recognizing these differences is key to avoiding misunderstandings and cultivating effective communication in interfaith relationships where different language and communication practices may exist.

3. Religion and Spirituality:
Religious beliefs play a central role in shaping cultural identity and influencing the worldviews of individuals. Respecting and appreciating different religious backgrounds is essential in interfaith relations. Open dialogue about religious practices, traditions and beliefs can create a platform for shared understanding and promote harmonious coexistence.

4. Time Orientation:
Cultures differ in their approach to time, with some emphasizing punctuality and efficiency (monochronic) while others favor flexibility and relationships over strict schedules (polychronic). Recognizing these differences is essential to avoid misunderstanding and frustration in cultural and interfaith relationships where different views of time may exist.

5. Social structures:

The way societies are organized, including family structures, social hierarchies, and gender roles, significantly influences cultural dynamics. In interfaith relationships, understanding and respecting these social structures helps to overcome potential challenges and build connections that transcend cultural and religious differences.

6. Cultural sensitivity and awareness:
Developing cultural sensitivity means being aware of and appreciating the differences that exist between individuals from different cultural and religious backgrounds. This awareness helps to avoid stereotypes and prejudices and promotes a more inclusive and respectful environment in cultural and interfaith relations.

7. Intercultural competence:
Intercultural competence includes the ability to navigate and communicate effectively across different cultures. In interfaith relationships, individuals with high intercultural competence can bridge gaps, facilitate understanding, and build

connections that transcend religious differences. This competence is built on knowledge, awareness and the ability to adapt to different cultural contexts.

8. Cultural adaptation and flexibility:

Cultural relationships often require adaptation and flexibility. Being open to accepting new customs, traditions and ways of thinking increases the quality of interactions. In interfaith relationships, this adaptability is especially crucial, as it allows individuals to navigate the intricacies of different religious practices and beliefs.

Orientation in the dimensions of culture is an integral part of supporting positive cultural and interreligious relations. It requires a commitment to understanding, respect and open communication. Embracing diversity and recognizing the richness it brings to relationships allows individuals to build connections that transcend cultural and religious boundaries. In a world characterized by increasing globalization and interconnectedness, the ability to navigate and appreciate diverse cultures is not only desirable, but also necessary to create a harmonious and inclusive global community.

2.2 Communication Styles Across Cultures

In our interconnected global society, cultural and interfaith relationships are becoming increasingly common, bringing together people from different backgrounds and communication styles. Successful orientation in these relationships requires a deep understanding of the dynamics of communication inherent in different cultures. Communication styles shaped by cultural nuances and religious beliefs play a key role in promoting mutual understanding and harmony.

Cultural influence on communication styles:
Cultures around the world exhibit different communication preferences, influenced by historical, social and economic factors. In high-context cultures such as Japan and many Middle Eastern countries, communication is often indirect and relies heavily on non-verbal cues. Understanding context is essential in such societies, as much of the message is conveyed through gestures, tone, and implied meanings.

On the other hand, low-context cultures, including those in North America and Western Europe, tend to favor explicit verbal communication. Clarity and directness are valued in these societies, and individuals often speak their minds without relying too much on non-verbal cues. Recognizing these differences is essential in cultural relations to avoid misinterpretations and promote effective communication.

Religious Influences on Communication Styles:
In interfaith relationships, religious beliefs can significantly shape communication styles. For example, cultures influenced by Islam often value humility, respect, and indirect communication. In contrast, some Christian cultures may emphasize openness and assertiveness in expressing thoughts and feelings. Awareness of these religious nuances is essential to creating an atmosphere of acceptance and understanding in interfaith relationships.

In addition, religious practices can affect the rhythm of daily life and communication patterns. For example, in Hindu cultures where joint family systems predominate, communication often extends beyond the nuclear family to include extended relatives. Understanding and respecting these practices is an integral part of building strong interfaith relationships.

Challenges and Opportunities:
While differences in communication styles across cultures and faiths can present challenges, they also present opportunities for personal growth and enrichment. Experience with different communication approaches allows individuals in these relationships to broaden their perspectives, develop empathy, and become more adaptive communicators.

However, misunderstandings can occur when communication expectations are not explicitly communicated and negotiated. It is essential for individuals in intercultural and interfaith relationships to engage in open dialogues about their communication preferences, recognizing and respecting the diversity that each person brings to the relationship.

Effective cross-cultural communication:
Building effective communication in cultural and interfaith relationships requires proactive efforts. Here are some strategies to improve understanding and bridge communication gaps:

1. Cultural Sensitivity: Develop cultural sensitivity by learning about your partner's cultural background, traditions, and communication norms. This knowledge provides a basis for empathy and helps avoid unintentional offense.

2. Active Listening: Develop active listening skills to understand the nuances in your partner's communication. This includes not only hearing the words, but also paying attention to tone, body language, and cultural context.

3. Open Communication: Create an environment where open communication is encouraged. Encourage your partner to express their thoughts and feelings, and be receptive to feedback without judgment.

4. Adaptability: Be adaptable in your communication style. While remaining authentic, be willing to adjust your communication approach to suit your partner's preferences when necessary.

5. Patience and Understanding: Be aware that misunderstandings may occur and patience is necessary. Instead of reacting impulsively, take the time to understand your partner's perspective and find common ground together.

Successful communication in intercultural and interreligious relations requires a nuanced understanding of different communication styles influenced by culture and religion. Embracing these differences as opportunities for growth and enrichment can lead to stronger, more resilient relationships. By actively engaging in open communication, cultivating empathy, and adapting to each other's styles, individuals can navigate the complexities of cross-cultural relationships with grace and mutual respect.

2.3 Cultural Sensitivity and Awareness

Cultural sensitivity and awareness play a key role in fostering healthy relationships, especially in the context of diverse cultural and interfaith interactions. In an increasingly interconnected world, individuals from different cultural backgrounds come together and bring unique perspectives, traditions and beliefs. Navigating these differences sensitively and consciously is essential to building strong connections and fostering mutual understanding.

Understanding Cultural Sensitivity:
Cultural sensitivity involves recognizing and respecting the diversity of cultures, values and norms. It goes beyond mere recognition, requiring an active effort to understand, appreciate and adapt to the customs and practices of others. In cultural and interreligious relations, this sensitivity serves as the basis for harmonious coexistence.

Awareness of cultural nuances:
Being culturally aware means being attuned to the nuances of different cultures. This awareness

extends to language, gestures and social customs. Misunderstandings can easily occur when individuals are unaware of the subtleties that define cultural interactions. For example, a seemingly innocuous gesture may have a different meaning in another culture, highlighting the importance of being aware of these nuances.

Communication as a bridge:

Effective communication is the cornerstone of cultural sensitivity. Clear and open dialogue allows individuals to express their thoughts and feelings, creating a bridge between different cultural and interfaith perspectives. Fostering an environment where individuals feel comfortable sharing their cultural backgrounds and beliefs without fear of judgment is essential in these relationships.

Respecting religious diversity:

Interfaith relationships add another layer of complexity as individuals from different religious backgrounds meet. Respect for religious diversity is paramount, requiring understanding and acceptance of different belief systems. Interfaith couples often face unique challenges, and cultural sensitivity plays a key role in managing these challenges with empathy and respect.

Celebrating Diversity:

Cultural sensitivity goes beyond tolerance; includes the celebration of diversity. Embracing the richness of different cultures and faiths contributes to a more open and harmonious society. Instead of viewing differences as obstacles, individuals in cultural and interfaith relationships can use their diversity to create a more vibrant and dynamic shared experience.

Challenges and Opportunities:

While cultural and interfaith relationships offer opportunities for growth and learning, they also present challenges. Conflicting traditions, social expectations and stereotypes can disrupt relationships. Cultural sensitivity becomes a tool to overcome these challenges by encouraging open communication and a willingness to learn from one another.

Education and Awareness Building:

Fostering cultural sensitivity requires ongoing education and awareness building. Schools, workplaces and communities can play a vital role in fostering an environment that values diversity. Educational programs, workshops, and cultural exchange initiatives can help individuals develop the skills needed to successfully navigate cultural and interfaith relationships.

Empathy and Perspective:

Empathy is the cornerstone of cultural sensitivity. Putting yourself in another person's shoes promotes a deeper understanding of their cultural and religious perspectives. This ability to see the world through someone else's eyes builds empathy, creating stronger bonds in cultural and interfaith relationships.

Cultural sensitivity and awareness are indispensable in the complex tapestry of cultural and interfaith relations. As individuals navigate the complexities of different environments, adopting these principles can lead to richer and more fulfilling connections. By fostering open communication, celebrating diversity and approaching differences with empathy, cultural and interfaith relationships can flourish and contribute to a more inclusive and connected global community.

2.4 Challenges and Strategies in Cross-Cultural Relationships

Intercultural relationships, especially those involving different cultural and interreligious backgrounds, bring both richness and complexity to the dynamics of human connection. Managing the challenges inherent in these relationships requires a deep understanding of cultural nuances, effective communication strategies, and a commitment to fostering mutual respect.

One of the main challenges in intercultural relations is the clash of cultural values and expectations. Individuals from different backgrounds may have conflicting beliefs, attitudes, and customs, leading to potential misunderstandings. For example, approaches to family dynamics, gender roles, and communication styles can vary greatly across cultures. In interfaith relationships, religious practices and traditions may differ, adding another layer of complexity.

Open and honest communication is paramount to addressing these challenges. Couples need to engage in thoughtful discussions about their cultural backgrounds and explore the values and traditions that shape their perspectives. This not only promotes mutual understanding, but also creates a basis for compromise and accommodation. Recognizing and respecting differences while finding common ground can strengthen a relationship and contribute to its longevity.

Language barriers also represent a significant obstacle in intercultural relations. Communication is the lifeblood of any relationship, and misunderstandings arising from language differences can lead to frustration and conflict. Partners may interpret expressions, tone or gestures differently, leading to unintended offense.

Strategies to overcome language barriers include language education initiatives for both partners. This not only facilitates smoother communication, but also demonstrates a commitment to understanding each other's cultural nuances. In addition, using a combination of languages and using non-verbal cues can improve understanding and bridge the communication gap.

In interfaith relations, the issue goes beyond language to include religious practices and beliefs. It is essential for partners to engage in respectful conversations about their faith and to recognize the importance of religious identity in shaping individual worldviews. Creating a framework for mutual acceptance and accommodation of religious differences can help prevent conflicts related to opposing views.

Another critical aspect of cross-cultural relationships is the potential influence of family and societal expectations. Families, especially in more traditional cultures, may have specific expectations regarding mate selection, marriage rituals, and family dynamics. Balancing these expectations with individual autonomy within the relationship requires careful negotiation.

Strategies for managing external expectations include setting clear boundaries and encouraging open communication within the relationship. Couples may need to have conversations with their families, emphasizing the strength of their bond and their commitment to building a future together. Educating family members about the richness that diversity brings to a relationship can also contribute to a more supportive environment.

Cultural celebrations and holidays provide opportunities for joy and connection, but they can also be a source of stress in cross-cultural relationships. Deciding which traditions to prioritize, especially in interfaith relationships, can lead to tension. Partners need to find a balance that respects the importance of each other's traditions while creating new rituals that have personal meaning for both.

Intercultural relationships, especially those involving different cultural and interreligious backgrounds, require deliberate efforts to overcome problems. Effective communication, mutual respect and a willingness to adapt are key strategies for building successful and fulfilling relationships. By embracing the richness of diversity and navigating complexity with empathy, couples can create a solid foundation for harmonious and lasting differences.

Chapter 3: Interfaith Dynamics: Unity in Diversity

Interfaith dynamics play a key role in promoting unity in diversity, especially in the context of cultural and interfaith relations. In a world marked by a rich tapestry of beliefs, traditions and customs, the intersection of different faiths and cultures presents both challenges and opportunities. Embracing the concept of "Unity in Diversity" becomes imperative to create harmonious societies that respect and celebrate the differences between individuals.

Cultural diversity is an inherent aspect of human societies, with each culture contributing unique perspectives, values, and practices. Similarly, religious diversity adds another layer to this complexity, shaping the worldview of individuals and influencing societal norms. Interaction between different cultures and faiths can be a source of enrichment, broadening perspectives and encouraging mutual understanding.

At the heart of interfaith dynamics is the recognition that, despite differing views, there are shared human values that form the basis for meaningful connections. These common traits, such as compassion, empathy, and the pursuit of justice, serve as bridges that connect people from different cultural and religious backgrounds. Recognizing these shared values creates a basis for dialogue and cooperation and fosters a sense of unity in the midst of diversity.

One of the key aspects of promoting unity in diversity is interfaith dialogue. This includes open and respectful conversations between individuals of different faiths that allow them to share their beliefs, practices and experiences. Interfaith dialogue provides a platform for learning, dispelling misconceptions and building relationships based on mutual respect. By engaging in meaningful conversations, individuals can discover common ground that unites them, transcending religious and cultural differences.

Education plays a key role in promoting interfaith dynamism and unity in diversity. Schools, universities and communities can implement curricula that emphasize the contribution of different cultures and religions and promote appreciation of diversity from an early age. Exposure to different perspectives can dispel stereotypes and prejudices and pave the way for a more inclusive society where individuals from different backgrounds coexist harmoniously.

In addition, interfaith initiatives that encourage collaborative projects and joint celebrations can contribute to a sense of unity. Festivals, community service projects and cultural events provide opportunities for people of different faiths to meet and foster a sense of belonging and shared humanity. These initiatives showcase the richness of cultural and religious diversity while emphasizing the interconnectedness of all individuals.

However, navigating interfaith dynamics requires addressing the potential challenges and conflicts that may arise. Misunderstandings, stereotypes, and historical tensions can impede progress toward unity in diversity. Addressing these issues includes promoting religious literacy, dispelling myths, and promoting open communication. Furthermore, fostering a culture of tolerance and acceptance is essential to creating a society where differences are celebrated rather than feared.

We can say that interreligious dynamics play a key role in shaping cultural and interreligious relations. Embracing the concept of unity in diversity requires a commitment to understanding, respect and dialogue. By recognizing shared human values, engaging in interfaith dialogue, promoting education, and addressing challenges head-on, societies can build bridges that connect individuals from different cultural and religious backgrounds. Ultimately, promoting unity in diversity contributes to the creation of more inclusive, harmonious and resilient communities.

3.1 Exploring Interfaith Relationships

In a world marked by diversity and globalization, the intersection of cultures and faiths is increasingly common. Interfaith relationships, where individuals from different religious backgrounds meet, offer a unique lens through which to explore the rich tapestry of human connections. This exploration becomes even more nuanced when cultural elements are woven into the fabric of these relationships, creating a dynamic interplay of traditions, values and beliefs.

Understanding Interfaith Relations:
Interfaith relationships often serve as bridges that connect diverse worlds and promote understanding and tolerance. These unions represent an opportunity for individuals to walk the delicate balance between maintaining their religious identity while embracing the diversity inherent in their partner's faith. Cultural nuances further enrich the experience as traditions and customs intertwine, creating a harmonious blend that reflects the couple's shared values.

Challenges and opportunities:
While interfaith relationships provide many opportunities for growth and mutual respect, they are not without challenges. Navigating different religious practices and customs requires open communication, empathy, and a willingness to learn. Cultural differences can manifest in various aspects, from food preferences to family dynamics, requiring compromise and a shared commitment to

create a unique identity that respects the origins of both partners.

Cultural sensitivity:

Cultural sensitivity is the cornerstone of successful interfaith relations. It means embracing the beauty of diversity without diluting one's own cultural heritage. Partners learn to appreciate the intricacies of each other's traditions and create an environment where both individuals can celebrate their respective cultural festivals, rituals and ceremonies. This mutual respect forms the basis for a resilient and inclusive relationship.

Raising children in an interreligious and intercultural environment:

One of the most pressing aspects of interfaith relations is the question of how to raise children in the context of different religious and cultural backgrounds. Couples often embark on a journey of learning and seek a middle ground that allows their children to appreciate the traditions of both parents. This process includes fostering an environment where children can ask questions, learn about different faiths, and develop their own understanding of spirituality and cultural identity.

Community and Social Dynamics:
Interfaith couples may experience varying degrees of acceptance in their communities. Some companies embrace diversity, while others can present challenges. A couple's ability to navigate these external dynamics depends on their internal foundation of trust and understanding. Over time, many interfaith couples become advocates of tolerance and acceptance, challenging societal norms and contributing to a larger conversation about unity in diversity.

Celebrating Unity in Diversity:
Ultimately, exploring interfaith relationships within cultural intersections is an opportunity to celebrate unity in diversity. It is a testament to the power of love and understanding to transcend religious and cultural boundaries. As society continues to evolve, these relationships serve as beacons of hope, proving that connections built on respect and

shared values can withstand the complexities of our modern, connected world.

Interfaith relations enriched by cultural intersections offer a profound insight into the possibilities of unity in the midst of diversity. As individuals navigate the delicate balance of honoring their roots while tapping into the richness of their partner backgrounds, they contribute to a global story of acceptance, understanding, and shared humanity. In a world where differences often divide, these relationships are a testament to the transformative power of love, respect, and a willingness to embark on a shared journey of exploration and growth.

3.2 Intersecting Values and Beliefs

In the tapestry of human relations, the intersection of values and beliefs plays a pivotal role, especially in the context of cultural and interreligious relations. Navigating the delicate balance between different belief systems requires openness, respect, and a willingness to embrace the rich tapestry of human diversity.

At the heart of cultural and interreligious relations lies the interplay of values that are dear to individuals. These values are often deeply rooted, shaped by upbringing, social norms and personal experiences. In an increasingly interconnected world, individuals from different cultural and religious backgrounds find themselves forming bonds that transcend traditional boundaries.

One of the key challenges in such relationships is negotiating different values and beliefs. While diversity can be a source of strength, it can also be a source of tension if not approached sensitively. Understanding and respecting the core values that shape an individual's identity are essential to building a harmonious union.

Cultural values, rooted in traditions, customs and social expectations, provide a framework for understanding how individuals relate to the world around them. In a multicultural relationship, partners may need to overcome differences in communication styles, family dynamics, and gender role expectations. This requires a willingness to learn from each other, to appreciate the uniqueness each brings to the relationship.

Similarly, interfaith relationships add another layer of complexity as individuals from different religious backgrounds meet. Religion often plays a central role in shaping personal values, ethical frameworks, and worldviews. Mutual respect for religious beliefs is crucial, as is the ability to engage in open and constructive dialogue about faith. Successful interfaith relationships often involve blending traditions, finding common ground, and fostering an environment of mutual acceptance.

The key to navigating the intersection of values and beliefs in cultural and interfaith relationships lies in effective communication. Open and honest conversations about individual values, expectations and aspirations are essential to building a solid foundation. This requires active listening and a genuine curiosity to understand the nuances of a partner's cultural or religious background.

Furthermore, compromise in these relationships becomes a valuable skill. Finding a middle ground that respects the values of both partners without compromising their individual identities is a delicate but necessary art. This may include creating new traditions that honor both cultural backgrounds, or finding ways to celebrate religious holidays together that embrace the richness of both worlds.

Education and awareness also play a vital role in promoting understanding in cultural and interfaith relations. Taking the time to learn about each other's cultural history, customs, and religious practices can deepen appreciation and reduce misunderstandings. This proactive approach demonstrates commitment to the relationship and recognition of the importance of shared knowledge.

In addition to individual efforts, the dynamics of these unions are influenced by social attitudes towards cultural and interreligious relations. A more inclusive and accepting social environment can provide much-needed support for couples navigating the tangle of different values and beliefs. Celebrating diversity at a societal level fosters an environment where individuals can freely express their identity without fear of judgment or discrimination.

The intersection of values and beliefs in cultural and interreligious relations requires a delicate dance of understanding, respect and compromise. Embracing diversity and actively engaging in open communication can turn potential challenges into opportunities for growth and enrichment. As individuals continue to connect across cultural and religious divides, the ability to navigate this intersection becomes a testament to the power of love and human connection.

3.3 Interfaith Challenges and Solutions

Interfaith challenges in cultural and interfaith relations are complex and often arise from the intersection of different belief systems, traditions and cultural backgrounds. Tackling these challenges requires a nuanced understanding of the issues at hand and a commitment to fostering mutual respect and understanding. In this survey, we will delve into the key challenges we face in interfaith relations and propose constructive solutions to promote harmony and cooperation.

One of the main challenges in interfaith relations is the clash of religious doctrines. Different belief systems may have conflicting principles and practices, leading to potential conflicts. This dissonance can manifest itself in various aspects of daily life, from rituals and ceremonies to moral and ethical values. Open communication is paramount to solving this problem. Couples and communities need to create a space for dialogue where individuals can express their beliefs without judgment. This facilitates a deeper understanding of each other's perspectives and fosters an environment of acceptance.

Cultural differences also contribute to the complexity of interfaith relations. Customs, traditions, and social norms can vary greatly, influencing everything from family dynamics to societal expectations. Building bridges between cultures requires an appreciation of diversity and a willingness to learn from one another. Learning about each other's cultural backgrounds can bridge gaps and dispel stereotypes. Encouraging shared experiences, such as participating in each other's cultural celebrations, can strengthen the bond between individuals and communities.

In many cases, individuals face external pressures from their respective religious or cultural communities, which can disrupt interfaith relations. Fear of judgment or ostracism can lead individuals to hide their relationships or conform to societal expectations. A broader societal shift towards tolerance and inclusiveness is needed to overcome this challenge. Religious and cultural leaders can play a key role in promoting acceptance and encouraging openness in their communities.

Interfaith relationships can also struggle with the question of how to raise children in the context of many religions. Determining what religious or cultural practices to incorporate into a child's upbringing can be a source of tension. The key to meeting this challenge is compromise and flexibility. Couples need to engage in honest conversations about their expectations and priorities and seek common ground that respects the heritage of both partners. It may also involve finding a middle ground that allows children to explore and appreciate both faiths.

In seeking solutions to these challenges, it is essential to recognize the shared values that often underlie different religions and cultures. Common principles such as compassion, love and justice can serve as a basis for building understanding. Interfaith initiatives that focus on joint community projects, charitable activities, and social justice can bring people together in meaningful ways and foster a sense of unity that transcends religious and cultural boundaries.

In addition, educational programs promoting religious and cultural literacy can contribute to breaking down stereotypes and promoting a more informed and tolerant society. Schools, community centers, and religious institutions can play a role in providing resources that increase understanding and appreciation for different cultures and faiths.

The challenges in interfaith relations in the context of culture are multifaceted and require a combination of open communication, education, and societal shifts toward greater acceptance. By promoting understanding, respecting diversity and promoting shared values, individuals and communities can navigate the complexities of interfaith relations and build a more inclusive and harmonious society.

3.4 Case Studies: Successful Interfaith Relationships

Interfaith relationships, where individuals from different religious backgrounds meet in love and partnership, are increasingly common in our diverse and interconnected world. The dynamics of these relationships often present unique challenges, but also offer profound opportunities for understanding, respect, and unity. Examining successful case studies of interfaith relationships provides valuable insights into the factors that contribute to their success, particularly in the context of cultural and religious diversity.

One notable case study of a successful interfaith relationship is the story of Sarah and Raj. Sarah, coming from a Christian background, and Raj, with a Hindu upbringing, navigated the complexities of intertwining their cultural and religious identities. What stood out on their journey was a commitment to open communication. They spent time discussing and learning about each other's faith, rituals and traditions. This not only fostered mutual understanding but also strengthened their bond by recognizing and respecting the richness of their respective cultural heritage.

Furthermore, successful interfaith relationships often emphasize shared values that transcend religious differences. In the case of Sarah and Raj, they found common ground in their commitment to compassion, kindness and social justice. By focusing on these shared principles, they were able to build a solid foundation for their relationship, enabling them to navigate the challenges that arose from their diverse religious backgrounds.

Another illuminating case study involves Fatima and David, a couple who exemplify the successful integration of Islam and Judaism into their relationship. Their key to success was embracing diversity within the family unit. They celebrated both Islamic and Jewish holidays and exposed their children to the richness of both traditions. This approach not only fostered an inclusive environment, but also instilled in their children a deep appreciation of cultural diversity and religious tolerance.

Flexibility and compromise play a key role in successful interfaith relations. Maya and Alejandro, a couple with Buddhist and agnostic backgrounds, showed how compromise can lead to the harmonious coexistence of different belief systems. They established the practice of taking turns in attending religious or cultural events. This flexibility allowed them to maintain their individual identities while actively participating in and supporting each other's traditions.

In addition, the support of the wider community is often key to the success of interfaith relations. In the case of Priya and James, who came from Sikh and Christian backgrounds, the acceptance and encouragement from their families and social circles went a long way in strengthening their relationship. The couple actively worked with both communities and fostered a sense of unity that transcended religious boundaries.

Successful interfaith relationships underscore the importance of education and awareness. Couples like Aisha and Michael, who converted to Islam and Buddhism, prioritized learning about each other's faith. Together they attended religious events, read sacred texts and engaged in thoughtful discussions. This commitment to ongoing education not only deepened their connection, but also allowed them to address potential misunderstandings before they became serious issues.

Examining successful case studies of interfaith relationships reveals common threads that contribute to their strength and resilience. Open communication, a focus on shared values, flexibility, compromise, community support and a commitment to education are key elements that pave the way for a harmonious and lasting partnership. As our world continues to embrace diversity, these case studies serve as beacons of inspiration, showing that love really can transcend cultural and religious differences.

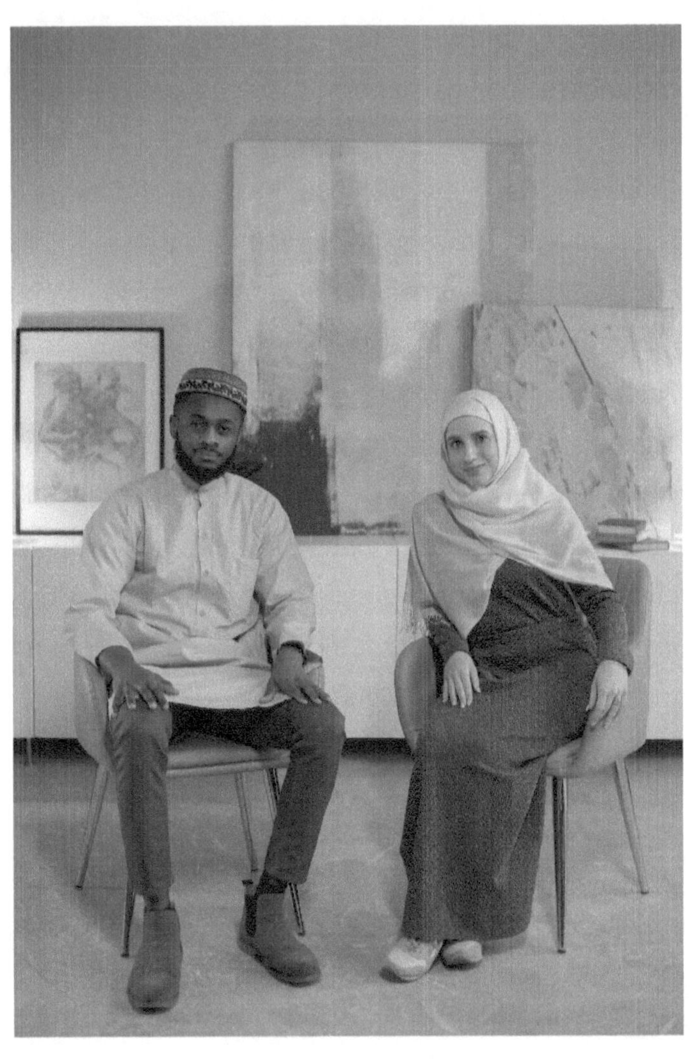

Chapter 4: Building Strong Cultural and Interfaith Connections

Building strong cultural and interfaith ties is essential to promote understanding, harmony and cooperation between different communities. In an increasingly interconnected world where people from different backgrounds coexist, it is essential to bridge the gaps that may exist between different cultures and faiths. This not only enriches the lives of individuals but also contributes to the overall well-being and prosperity of society.

Cultural and interreligious relations are dynamic and multifaceted, influenced by historical, social and political factors. Appreciating the richness and diversity that each culture and faith brings is essential to building strong relationships. This includes overcoming stereotypes and actively seeking to understand the nuances that shape the beliefs and practices of different communities.

One of the key aspects of building strong cultural and interfaith ties is fostering open communication. Creating a platform for dialogue allows individuals from different backgrounds to share their experiences, values and traditions. This exchange of perspectives can dispel misconceptions, reduce prejudice, and promote mutual respect. In a world where misinformation can spread quickly, creating space for honest and constructive conversations becomes a powerful tool in cultivating understanding.

Education plays a key role in this process. Incorporating cultural and interfaith studies into the curriculum helps equip individuals with the knowledge and skills needed to navigate a globalized world. By learning about the customs, history, and belief systems of others, individuals can develop a broader perspective that transcends cultural and religious boundaries. This educational approach promotes empathy, tolerance and a sense of shared humanity.

Interfaith dialogue is a specific aspect of this broader conversation. It involves individuals from different religious backgrounds coming together to explore the commonalities and differences in their religious traditions. Interfaith dialogue promotes religious literacy and understanding and emphasizes the universal values shared by many religions. This not only builds bridges between religious communities, but also contributes to the overall fabric of social cohesion.

Building strong cultural and interfaith ties also requires addressing issues that may arise as a result of cultural misunderstandings or religious differences. Conflict resolution mechanisms that include cultural sensitivity and respect for different beliefs are essential. This includes developing skills in intercultural communication and conflict mediation, enabling communities to deal with differences peacefully.

Another key part of strengthening cultural and interfaith ties is promoting inclusivity. Inclusive practices ensure that individuals from all cultural and religious backgrounds feel welcome and valued in diverse social settings. This includes creating an environment that celebrates diversity and actively works against discrimination. In workplaces, educational institutions and public spaces, inclusiveness promotes a sense of belonging and unity among people from different backgrounds.

Art and media also play an important role in building cultural and interfaith ties. Through literature, music, film, and other forms of artistic expression, people can gain insight into the perspectives and experiences of others. Cultural and interfaith themes in the arts provide a powerful medium for promoting understanding and empathy, overcoming language and cultural barriers.

Community involvement is a practical way to realize the ideals of building strong cultural and interfaith ties. Participation in cultural events, religious celebrations and community initiatives enables individuals to actively experience and appreciate the diversity around them. This hands-on approach fosters a sense of shared humanity and helps break down barriers that may exist between different cultural and religious groups.

Governments and policy makers also play a key role in promoting cultural and interfaith ties. Policies that promote diversity, multiculturalism and religious freedom contribute to creating inclusive societies. By recognizing and appreciating the contributions of all communities, governments can set the tone for promoting harmony and cooperation among diverse populations.

Building strong cultural and interfaith ties is a continuous and collective effort involving individuals, communities, educational institutions, governments and various organizations. Embracing diversity, promoting open communication, promoting education and actively engaging in intercultural and interreligious dialogue are essential steps to creating a world where people from different backgrounds coexist harmoniously. Ultimately, the power of these connections lies in recognizing our shared humanity and celebrating the unique contributions each culture and faith makes to the global tapestry of human experience.

4.1 Fostering Mutual Respect and Understanding

Promoting mutual respect and understanding in cultural and interreligious relations

In an increasingly connected world, the tapestry of human diversity is more prominent than ever. Cultural and interfaith relations have become an integral part of our global society, bringing together individuals from different backgrounds, beliefs and traditions. However, with this diversity comes the need to foster mutual respect and understanding to ensure harmonious coexistence. In navigating the complex nuances of cultural and interfaith relations, embracing diversity becomes not only a choice but a fundamental commitment to build bridges rather than walls.

The basis of successful cultural and interreligious relations is mutual respect. Respect is the cornerstone upon which understanding is built, creating a foundation that allows individuals to appreciate and acknowledge the differences that make each person unique. It includes recognizing the intrinsic value of different perspectives, traditions and beliefs, fostering an environment where everyone feels seen, heard and valued.

One of the key aspects of cultivating mutual respect is active listening. In the context of cultural and interfaith relations, this means paying genuine attention to the experiences, beliefs and narratives of others. By listening with an open heart and mind, individuals can gain insight into different worldviews and gain a deeper understanding of the cultural and religious tapestry that shapes one's identity.

In addition, education plays a key role in promoting mutual respect and understanding. Learning about the customs, traditions and history of different cultures and faiths not only broadens knowledge but also develops empathy. Educational initiatives that promote cultural competence and interfaith understanding can bridge gaps in awareness, dispel stereotypes and misconceptions that can lead to prejudice or discrimination.

Embracing cultural humility is another essential element in fostering healthy relationships from diverse backgrounds. Cultural humility involves a commitment to self-reflection, acknowledging that one's cultural lens may limit one's understanding of others. It encourages individuals to approach interactions with a sense of curiosity and a willingness to learn, creating an environment where cultural exchange can thrive.

In the field of interfaith relations, dialogue becomes a powerful tool for building bridges. Open and respectful conversations about religious belief, practice and values can dispel misunderstandings and foster a deeper appreciation of the diversity of religious traditions. Interfaith dialogue promotes the idea that shared values and common goals can exist across religious boundaries and emphasizes the universal principles that bind humanity together.

In addition to dialogue, participation in shared experiences and celebrations can strengthen bonds between individuals of different cultures and faiths. Celebrating cultural festivals, participating in religious ceremonies, or participating in community events provides an opportunity for mutual respect to blossom organically. Shared experiences create common ground and foster a sense of unity that transcends cultural and religious differences.

However, problems can arise in cultural and interreligious relations, and their resolution requires patience, empathy and a determination to find common ground. Conflict resolution becomes an essential skill in handling disagreements or misunderstandings and ensures that differences do not grow into barriers that divide communities.

Fostering mutual respect and understanding in cultural and interfaith relations is an ongoing process that requires commitment, education and an open mind. Embracing diversity, active listening, engaging in dialogue and participating in shared experiences all contribute to the cultivation of a harmonious and inclusive society. In a world where cultural and interfaith interactions are increasingly prevalent, fostering mutual respect becomes not only a choice, but a shared responsibility to build a more connected and compassionate global community.

4.2 Interfaith Dialogue and Collaboration

Interfaith dialogue and cooperation play a vital role in promoting understanding, tolerance and harmony between different cultural and religious communities. In an age marked by globalization and interconnectedness, the need for effective communication and cooperation between different religions and cultures is more important than ever. This contextual survey will delve into the importance of interfaith dialogue and cooperation in the field of cultural and interfaith relations and illuminate the positive impact they can have on individuals and society as a whole.

At its core, interfaith dialogue is a dynamic process of communication that crosses religious boundaries and encourages individuals from different faith traditions to engage in open and respectful conversations. This dialogue serves as a bridge, connecting people who may hold different beliefs, practices and cultural backgrounds. It offers a platform for individuals to share their experiences, values and perspectives, creating a rich tapestry of diversity that contributes to the cultural mosaic of our global society.

One of the fundamental advantages of interreligious dialogue is the promotion of mutual understanding. Through open and honest conversations, participants gain insight into others' beliefs and practices, dispelling misconceptions and stereotypes that can be divisive. This understanding becomes a powerful tool in breaking down barriers, fostering empathy and cultivating a sense of unity in the midst of diversity.

Interwoven with interfaith dialogue, cultural relations create a space where individuals can appreciate the richness of diverse traditions. By recognizing the commonalities that unite different cultures, people can celebrate their shared humanity while respecting the unique aspects that make each culture different. This celebration of diversity not only enriches personal experiences, but also contributes to creating a more inclusive and tolerant society.

Interfaith cooperation goes beyond dialogue and involves joint efforts to address common challenges and promote shared values. Whether it's solving social problems, advocating for human rights, or engaging in community service, joint initiatives bring individuals of different faiths together to work for the common good. This shared commitment fosters a sense of solidarity and shows that diverse communities can overcome challenges when they come together for a common purpose.

In addition, interfaith cooperation has the potential to play a key role in conflict resolution and peace promotion. In regions where religious and cultural differences are a source of tension, joint efforts can serve as a catalyst for reconciliation. Through joint projects, shared initiatives and joint problem solving, communities can build trust and work to create a more harmonious coexistence.

Education plays a key role in developing interreligious dialogue and cooperation. Implementing educational programs that promote religious literacy and cultural understanding helps dispel ignorance and prejudice. By fostering an environment where individuals can learn about different religions and cultures, educational institutions contribute to the development of open-minded and informed citizens who are better equipped to engage in meaningful interfaith dialogue.

Governments, NGOs and religious institutions all have roles to play in promoting and promoting interfaith dialogue and cooperation. Policies that promote inclusivity, protect religious freedom, and support initiatives aimed at promoting interfaith understanding contribute to creating a more tolerant and harmonious society.

Interfaith dialogue and cooperation serve as powerful tools in building bridges across different cultures and religions. By fostering mutual understanding, celebrating diversity, and fostering collaborative efforts, these practices contribute to the creation of a more inclusive and harmonious global community. In a world where cultural and interreligious relations are increasingly interconnected, investing in these dialogues becomes not only a necessity, but also a beacon of hope for a future characterized by unity in diversity.

4.3 Celebrating Cultural and Religious Diversity

In an increasingly interconnected world, the celebration of cultural and religious diversity has become paramount, especially in the context of cultural and interfaith relations. These relationships are a testament to the rich tapestry of human experience and show the beauty that arises when individuals from different cultural and religious backgrounds come together in harmony.

At the heart of celebrating cultural and religious diversity is the recognition that each individual brings a unique set of traditions, beliefs and values to the table. Embracing this diversity fosters an environment of mutual respect and understanding. Cultural and interfaith relationships provide a platform for people to learn from each other and enrich their lives with perspectives that transcend their own cultural or religious upbringing.

One of the key elements in celebrating diversity is the recognition of different cultural practices. Whether celebrating festivals, traditional ceremonies or daily rituals, every cultural aspect contributes to the mosaic of experiences. In cultural and interreligious relationships, partners have the opportunity to participate in and appreciate the customs of their significant other. This not only strengthens the bond between individuals, but also creates a shared space where both partners can freely express their cultural identity.

In addition, cultural and interreligious relations often lead to the creation of a unique mixture of traditions. Couples navigate the delicate balance of incorporating aspects from each other's backgrounds to create a hybrid cultural identity that reflects the amalgamation of diverse influences. This synthesis of traditions serves as a testament to the adaptability and resilience of love in crossing cultural and religious boundaries.

Religious diversity in cultural and interfaith relations presents its own set of opportunities and challenges. However, it is essential to see these differences as a source of enrichment rather than division. Interfaith couples often find themselves in an open and respectful dialogue about their beliefs, which fosters a deeper understanding of their partner's spiritual journey. This process not only strengthens the emotional connection between individuals, but also cultivates an environment where different religious perspectives are valued.

Navigating religious diversity in a relationship requires commitment, communication, and a willingness to learn from each other. Interfaith couples often find common ground in shared values, ethical principles, and universal aspects of their faith. Celebrating religious diversity in these relationships involves creating a supportive environment where both partners can practice their beliefs without fear of judgment or compromise.

Education plays a key role in celebrating cultural and religious diversity in cultural and interfaith relations. Learning about each other's cultural heritage and religious background not only deepens understanding, but also removes stereotypes and prejudices. This educational aspect extends beyond the couple themselves to their families, friends and communities, promoting a wider acceptance of diverse relationships.

At the societal level, celebrating cultural and religious diversity in relationships contributes to a broader narrative of inclusivity. It challenges stereotypes and prejudices that may exist in communities and promotes the idea that love knows no cultural or religious boundaries. As cultural and interfaith relationships become more visible and accepted, they serve as powerful examples of unity in diversity and encourage others to embrace and celebrate differences.

However, it is important to note that the celebration of cultural and religious diversity in intercultural and interfaith relations is not without problems. Misunderstandings, social pressure, and outside judgments can create obstacles for couples navigating these diverse relationships. It takes resilience and determination to overcome these challenges, emphasizing the importance of open communication, mutual respect and a shared vision for the future.

Celebrating cultural and religious diversity in cultural and interfaith relations is a multifaceted path that involves accepting differences, promoting understanding, and creating a space where love can flourish despite a diverse environment. These relationships serve as beacons of unity in diversity, challenging societal norms and promoting a world where individuals are valued for who they are, regardless of their cultural or religious affiliation. As we continue to navigate an ever-evolving global environment, celebrating cultural and religious diversity in relationships becomes not only a choice, but a collective responsibility to build a more inclusive and compassionate world.

4.4 Nurturing Inclusivity in Communities

In an ever-changing and interconnected world, the importance of cultivating inclusivity within communities cannot be overstated. As diverse cultures and faiths coexist, fostering a sense of unity and understanding becomes paramount. This journey towards inclusivity involves embracing the richness of diversity, particularly in the realm of cultural and interfaith relationships.

Embracing Cultural Diversity:
Cultural diversity is the tapestry that weaves together the fabric of our global society. Communities are composed of individuals with unique traditions, customs, and histories. Nurturing inclusivity in this context involves celebrating these differences, recognizing them as valuable contributions that enrich the collective experience.
One way to promote cultural inclusivity is through educational initiatives. Workshops, events, and cultural exchange programs can provide community members with opportunities to learn about various

cultures firsthand. This not only breaks down stereotypes but also fosters an environment where curiosity replaces ignorance, paving the way for deeper understanding and acceptance.

Community leaders play a crucial role in setting the tone for inclusivity. They can actively promote diverse cultural events, encourage representation in decision-making processes, and create spaces where different cultural perspectives are acknowledged and respected. By fostering an atmosphere that values and appreciates cultural differences, communities can become more cohesive and harmonious.

Bridging Interfaith Relationships:
Interfaith relationships bring another layer of complexity to the tapestry of diversity. Different religious beliefs often coexist within communities, requiring a delicate balance of respect and understanding. Nurturing inclusivity in the context of interfaith relationships involves building bridges between various religious communities and fostering dialogue.

Interfaith dialogue can take many forms, from organized discussions to collaborative community projects. Engaging in open and respectful conversations allows individuals from different faith backgrounds to share their beliefs, dispel misconceptions, and find common ground. It is through this shared understanding that the foundations of a truly inclusive community are laid. Educational initiatives also play a crucial role in fostering inclusivity among diverse faiths. Schools, community centers, and religious institutions can organize seminars or workshops that provide insights into different belief systems. This not only promotes religious literacy but also dispels stereotypes, fostering an environment of tolerance and acceptance.

Leadership and Community Initiatives:
Leadership within a community is pivotal in shaping its values and priorities. Leaders who actively champion inclusivity set a positive example for others to follow. They can establish policies that promote diversity, ensure representation in decision-making bodies, and allocate resources to

support initiatives that celebrate different cultures and faiths.

Community initiatives that bring people together across cultural and religious lines strengthen the bonds that unite us. Festivals that showcase diverse traditions, service projects that involve members of various faiths working side by side, and collaborative cultural celebrations can create a sense of unity that transcends individual differences.

Moreover, establishing interfaith councils or committees within communities can provide a structured platform for ongoing dialogue and collaboration. These groups can address issues related to religious tolerance, promote understanding, and serve as mediators in times of potential conflict, contributing to the overall harmony of the community.

Challenges and Opportunities:

Nurturing inclusivity in communities, especially in the context of cultural and interfaith relationships, is not without its challenges. Misunderstandings, biases, and historical tensions may pose obstacles along the way. However, these challenges present opportunities for growth and transformation.

Addressing stereotypes and prejudices requires ongoing education and dialogue. Community members must be willing to confront their own biases and be open to learning from one another. Through this process, individuals can develop a deeper appreciation for the diversity within their community and recognize the common humanity that binds them together.

Nurturing inclusivity in communities with a focus on cultural and interfaith relationships is a multifaceted endeavor that requires commitment, education, and leadership. By celebrating cultural diversity, fostering interfaith dialogue, and implementing inclusive policies and initiatives, communities can create environments where every individual feels valued and respected. In doing so, they not only strengthen their social fabric but also contribute to a more interconnected and harmonious world.

CONCLUSION

In conclusion, cultural and interfaith relationships are invaluable assets that contribute to the rich tapestry of our global society. As we navigate the complexity of a connected world, it is becoming increasingly clear that fostering understanding, respect and appreciation for different cultures and faiths is not just a choice, but a necessity.

These relationships serve as bridges that span the gaps created by ignorance and prejudice. By embracing the beauty of our differences, we pave the way for a harmonious coexistence that transcends the boundaries of nationality, ethnicity, and religion. The tapestry of human experience is woven with threads of myriad hues, each representing a unique cultural or religious tradition. It is in the interweaving of these threads that we discover the true masterpiece that is our shared humanity.

In addition, cultural and interfaith relationships offer a profound opportunity for personal growth.

Working with individuals from diverse backgrounds encourages us to broaden our perspectives, challenge assumptions, and broaden our horizons. It is through this process of mutual learning and exchange that we develop the resilience and adaptability needed to thrive in an ever-changing global environment.

In addition, these relationships play a key role in eliminating stereotypes and refuting misconceptions that often arise from ignorance. By interacting with individuals from different cultural and religious backgrounds, we challenge preconceived notions and confront the humanity that unites us all. This in turn contributes to creating a more inclusive and tolerant society where the richness of diversity is celebrated rather than feared.

In the context of interfaith relations, the potential for building bridges of understanding is particularly significant. As the world grapples with religious tensions, prejudices and conflicts, fostering connections between people of different faiths becomes an urgent imperative. Through dialogue, shared experiences and a commitment to finding common ground, interfaith relationships have the power to break down barriers and promote a culture of peace and acceptance.

Furthermore, children born from cultural and interfaith unions embody the blending of different heritages and become living testimonies of the possibility of unity in diversity. These individuals often navigate the complexities of identity with a unique perspective and act as ambassadors for cultural understanding in a world that urgently needs it. Their very existence challenges the notion of fixed cultural and religious boundaries and paves the way for a more connected and compassionate future.

We can say that the benefits of cultural and interreligious relations are diverse. They improve our collective understanding, promote personal growth, break down stereotypes and contribute to building a more inclusive and tolerant global society. As we face the challenges of the 21st century, it is imperative that we recognize the transformative potential of these relationships and actively work to embrace the diversity that defines us as a species. Only through such collective efforts can we hope to build a world where cultural and interfaith relationships are not only accepted but celebrated as a cornerstone of our shared human experience

.

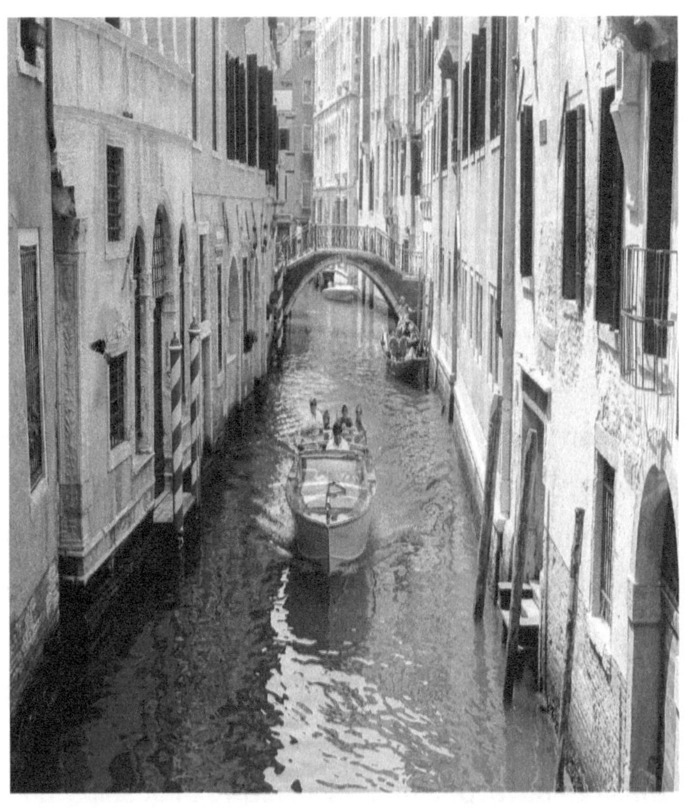